Black Women & Hair Loss

How To Stop Losing Our Hair & Gain Massive Hair Growth

by

Sabrina R Perkins

Seriouslynatural.org
naturalhairforbeginners.com

Black women are more prone to hair loss. Learn why and how to stop this vicious cycle.

Contents

Consult a professional

More Resources
Seriously Natural
Natural Hair For Beginners
How To Stop Hair Loss in Women□

Dedication

I have to dedicate this book to a few amazing people who directly encouraged me to finally put my pen to paper. I must dedicate this book to my mother, Gloria Richmond, for encouraging me to write professionally ever since I wrote my first story at the tender age of 7 years old. Love you mommy!

I also must dedicate this book to my best friend, husband and partner in crime, Matthew. I love you, and appreciate you believing in me and making sure I was always taken care of.

Introduction

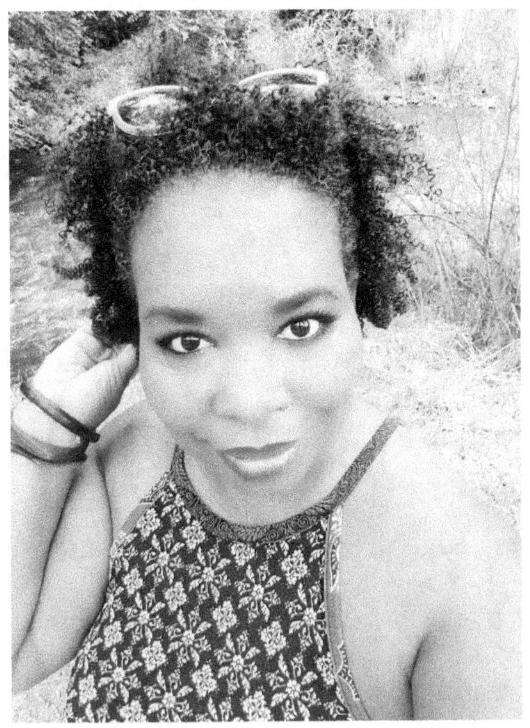

Welcome to How To Black Women & Hair Loss by me, Sabrina R Perkins, a natural hair and beauty blogger with two successful blogs, **seriouslynatural.org** and **naturalhairforbeginners.com**

This informative book is a quick and easy tool for not just stopping hair loss for Black women, but to understanding what it is and how to defeat it successfully. All too often Black women are being silent on hair loss and it's time to open our mouths for help and gain solid and accurate knowledge. Time to regain our healthy strands and beautiful hair.

Thinning edges, resorting to weaves and wigs for length or severe breakage does not have to be your reality and know that neglecting the problem will only make it worse. I'm so glad you decided to get the right knowledge to stop this cycle! So, now it's time to learn how to win against hair loss with this resourceful book.

Sabrina

Black Women & Hair Loss

How To Stop Losing Our Hair & Gain Massive Hair Growth

Chapter 1: What Is Hair Loss?

Believed to affect mostly men but can and does affect women, hair loss is defined as:

> "Hair loss is the thinning of hair on the scalp. The medical term for hair loss is alopecia. Alopecia can be temporary or permanent. The most common form of hair loss occurs gradually and is referred to as "androgenetic alopecia," meaning that a combination of hormones (androgens are male hormones) and heredity (genetics) is needed to develop the condition. Other types of hair loss include

alopecia areata (patches of baldness that usually grow back), telogen effluvium (rapid shedding after childbirth, fever, or sudden weight loss); and traction alopecia (thinning from tight braids or ponytails)."

This can be very distressing to many men and women who suffer from hair loss and while most women feel alone when suffering from hair loss, there are millions of women who will have some sort of hair loss during their lifetime. There are diverse types of hair loss so do not assume you are suffering from only one kind or that it will just go away. We have created this book so that you not only understand

hair loss but how to determine what kind,
how to stop it and how to create a healthy
environment for your hair to grow and
thrive.

Chapter 2: Why Do Black Women Suffer MORE From Hair Loss?

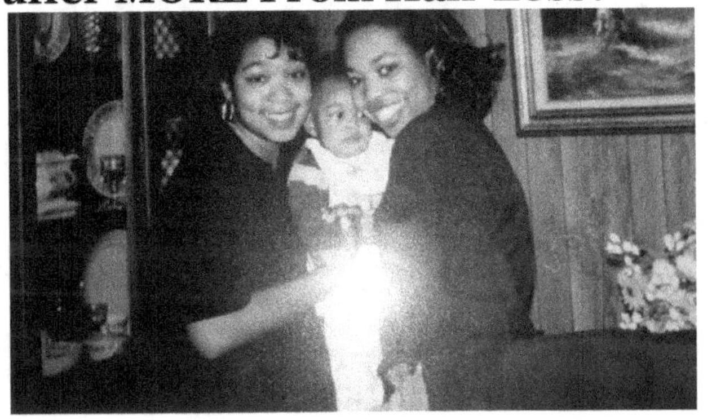

Hair loss is not just a problem for men as women make up 40% of American hair loss sufferers according to the American Hair Loss Association. Honestly, many women are suffering in silence and this devastating problem is no more felt harder than in the African American community.

A study published in 2016 and presented at the American Academy of Dermatology's 74th

Annual meeting showed alarming concerns for Black women. The study showed that Black women were more prone to hair loss and even more alarming was the fact that we are less likely to seek professional help to rectify the problem.

The cause for most of the hair loss for black women is a condition called Central Centrifugal Cicatricial Alopecia (CCCA) which is a disorder that causes inflammation and destruction to the hair follicles, can cause scarring and even permanent hair loss. This vital and alarming information was provided by Dr. Lenzy, a Board-certified dermatologist and clinical associate at University of Connecticut, Farmington, Conn.

Dr. Lenzy, along with other experts believe hair loss is a genetic disposition among black women and they are increasing the risk of hair loss by practicing damaging hair styling techniques like braids, chemical relaxing, and wearing weaves. Out of 5,594 black women who were part of the study and survey, almost 50% reported hair loss on the crown of their head and 81.4% of those women never sought any kind of help from a physician or dermatologist.

In another study during the same year, a consumer survey conducted by Keranique® – the Women's Hair Growth Experts™ sheds light on the alarming numbers of American women who have experienced hair loss. According to the survey:

- Nearly 40% of U.S. women 18+ have noticed signs of hair loss or thinning

- Over 50% of US women 58 or older have experienced it

- That number jumps to over 60% for women age 65+

- These signs include: a widening part, hair being thinner than it used to be, significant signs of overall hair loss, and seeing through to the scalp where they couldn't before especially in the temples or at the crown of the head.

Who is at risk?

Research indicates women in one or more of these 3 categories are more susceptible to hair loss and thinning:

- Women are 97% more likely (almost twice as likely) to experience signs of hair loss if they have a relative with hair loss compared to those who don't, and 61% of women who have relatives with hair loss are experiencing symptoms of hair loss.

- Women who have had chemical treatments are 71% more likely to experience hair loss than those who have not, and over half (58%) of women who have had chemical treatments are experiencing signs of hair loss.

- Women who have been ill or taking medicine are 81% more likely to suffer from hair loss and thinning than those who have not, and over half (58%) of women who have been ill or taking medicine are experiencing signs of hair loss.

- And many could be at risk for future issues. 62% of women have noticed changes to their hair just in the past year.

Why so many? Well, a few factors including unhealthy hair habits, stress, and lack of seeking help are all reasons for such devastating numbers. Ways to beat this are enlisting good hair habits with healthy hair education, living a healthier lifestyle, and seeking professional help from a physician, dermatologist or a trichologist are all excellent ways to combat the problem.

I even reached out to professional hairstylists for her take on this growing problem. Janeise Alexander, owner of J'Das Studio For Hair in Oakland, CA says many clients of hers experience hair follicle trauma.

"Tension from braids and twists can and does cause permanent follicle damage, especially to the lanugo (baby) hair around the perimeter of the head." She adds, "Chemicals such as relaxers and colors can also cause damage if the service isn't administered properly. Applying protection cream to the lanugo hair and scalp is a Must. Also, Neutralization and plenty of rinsing will help to remove all traces of the chemical."

In a nutshell, this is a problem that too few Black women are discussing or even thinking about. There is no help by trying to ignore the problem and we are here to change the narrative by giving sound advice to fix the problem of hair loss in Black Women.

Chapter 3: How Black Women Can Effectively Stop Hair Loss

No, this does not have to be our burden to bear. We can successfully stop hair loss and without enlisting expensive methods. Here are some simple, yet effective ways to stop the vicious cycle of hair loss and low hair growth for Black Women.

Limit or Lay Off the Chemicals

For many women, they don't even realize that they are causing their own hair loss because of poor hair etiquette. Some of the prettiest hairstyles are creating the most hair and scalp harm or trauma. Using chemicals for coloring and straightening break down the bonds of hair and damage the strands. You must rebuild the hair with protein and moisturizing products, but to keep using these types of products, can only keep damaging your strands.

To my Relaxed Black Women

I am not trying to sway anyone into to going natural as some women are just not interested or ready to take the plunge. Just know that many black women have incurred damaged hair and scalp because of those straightening chemicals and have found ways to straighten hair without their use. If you are dealing with hair loss and still want to stay relaxed, enlist the help of a professional hairstylist and/or Trichologist to make sure you are doing everything you can to fix the problem.

Lay off The Heat!

Another problem is using too much heat. Black women have been applying heat to our hair for decades, but we've been paying a hefty price for it from heat damage to severe dryness. Our desire for straight hair has been less than kind to our delicate tresses and the best way to change our unhealthy habits is to be fully aware of what we are using. As we back away from harmful hair care practices such as direct heat let's discuss what the two terms mean.

What is direct heat?

Heat from an appliance that is directly touching the hair for drying the hair or straightening the natural curl or coil of the hair texture. Examples of typical direct heat styling tools are:

- Flat Iron
- Blow-dryer (without a diffuser)

- Hot Comb

These tools although convenient, are harsh on the hair and dry it out or break the strands. The much-needed moisture our hair needs is depleted. They also create heat damage. Heat damage is hair that has had heat styling tools set on temperatures too high, too long, passed over too many times (or all of the above) and the hair loses its natural elasticity.

This damages the hair shaft and changes its original curl, coil or kink which is irreversible. We should be using direct heat sparingly (once a month or less) as even one application of direct heat can cause heat damage. If using direct heat, make sure to use a heat protectant and preferably one with silicones as silicones create a barrier around the hair to protect it from the heat styling tool.

What is Indirect Heat?

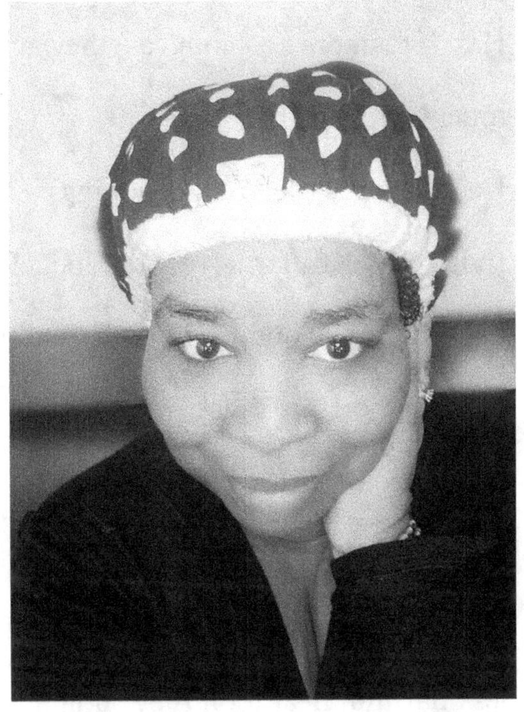

Indirect heat is far less harmful and beneficial in many applications. Their benefits usually come in the form of increasing moisture to the hair or drying hair safely. Examples of indirect styling tools are:

- Hooded Dryers

- Soft-bonnet dryers

- Hair Steamers (as long as they are not touching the hair)

- Heating Caps (deep conditioning)

- Indirect heat harnesses the benefits of heat for deep conditioning, drying hair or adding moisture back into the strands. This is done without whisking away hair's moisture or breaking the hair off by drying it out to death. Despite being a far less harmful heat tool, they should still be used on the lowest setting possible for the task.

Tips On Using Heat

No one is saying NEVER use direct heat. Just be smart about it and know this should not be an everyday or even every week practice.

- Always use the lowest setting

- Do not use direct heat often

- Always use a heat protectant

- Do not use direct heat on damaged hair (it will only make it worse)

- Do use moisturizing products from shampoos to conditioners to stylers to beef up your hair's moisture as direct heat tends to dry it out.

Ginger

Many of us know the benefits of a ginger, and some of us even enjoy a cup of ginger herbal tea_. This wonderful natural root has lots of uses in the culinary world, but few of us are probably aware that ginger also has many beauty benefits. This root is part of the Zingiberaceae family, along with cardamom and turmeric. It is commonly produced in India, Jamaica, Fiji, Indonesia, and Australia. From face masks to moisturizers, people have been applying this potent spice to their skin and hair for centuries.

One of the best things about ginger when it comes to beauty is its effect on hair. If you are one of the many people currently suffering from hair loss it may be a useful thing to try. In this article we give you the lowdown on how to use ginger to fight thinning and hair loss. Whether you have long, straight locks or gorgeous curls like 4a hair, ginger has a lot to offer. Ginger has a range of benefits for the scalp, roots and ends of hair, from stopping thinning to increasing blood flow and giving the hair much needed minerals. Here's an easy to do hair growth mask using ginger.

Ginger + Coconut Oil Hair Growth Mask

Ingredients:

1 Tbsp. finely grated Ginger

2 Tbsp. warmed slightly Coconut oil or Sesame oil

Cheesecloth or Muslin cloth

Method:

Blend the ginger into a fine paste before squeezing out the juice the cheesecloth or muslin cloth. Set the ginger juice to the side as you will be using it later. Combine the squeezed-out

ginger and coconut oil together until well mixed.
Add the ginger juice and still well.

How to use:

Use before washing hair by massaging the mixture into your scalp well. Cover with a plastic cap and leave in for at least one hour. Wash out with shampoo and style as usual.

Natural Oils

Natural oils, both essential and carrier hold a host of components that fight hair loss and even stimulate hair growth. Here is a list of some of the best natural oils for fighting hair loss.

Coconut Oil

Coconut oil contains Lauric acid which fights off various bacteria and fungi that can be found on the irritated scalps. Infections of the scalp can cause a significant amount of hair fall, as the follicles shed as they become swollen and irritated. Coconut oil is also known as the only oil that can fully penetrate the hair follicle, rebuilding it from the inside out and reducing the likelihood of unnecessary damage.

Olive Oil

Often used for cooking and salad dressings, olive oil is one of the most common household oils that can be found. Not only does it make a great vinaigrette, but it also contains an impressive amount of vitamin E and other monounsaturated fatty acids that promote hair growth and reduce hair fall. Of course, the more expensive and pure the olive oil is, the more vitamins and nutrient it will contain, so you may need to pay a pretty penny if you're looking for the top-notch results.

Castor Oil

Aside from causing an impressive "internal cleansing" ingredient, this oil also contains hair growth and regeneration properties. The oil's triglycerides of ricinoleic acid makes it anti-fungal, anti-bacterial and anti-inflammatory, which are all important components that are needed to both combat and prevent scalp infections, fungi and unhealthy bacteria. The restorative properties of castor oil strengthen the roots of the hair, therefore reducing shedding, while also causing new hairs to grow in quick, thick, and much healthier. Many women are finding the best way to regrow edges is by using Jamaican Black Castor Oil for scalp massages.

Check out this super popular hair stimulating hair mask using castor oil.

Castor, Mustard & Olive Oil Hair Growth Mask

<u>What you need:</u>

2 tbsp. castor oil

1 tbsp. mustard oil

1 tbsp. olive oil

<u>Method:</u>

Mix all three oils in a small bowl. Apply mixture to hair (also massage into scalp) and cover with shower cap or towel. Leave in at least for one hour before washing out with a gentle shampoo.

Lavender Oil

Lavender oil is stimulating, meaning that it increases circulation to the scalp. Not only does that encourage new hair growth, but it also provides much needed nutrients and oxygen to the roots of the hair, which makes the root stronger and reduces the amount of shedding. This oil also combats against nits and lice, which is something else that can lead to hair fall. Much like its counterparts, it also contains antibacterial properties that wards off infections, fungi and unwanted bacteria.

Sweet Almond Oil

Almond oil is known to be a natural "moisturizer" due to its softening properties. Containing Vitamins E and D, along a host of other minerals such as calcium and magnesium, makes almond oil one of the only oils that can prevent the hair from drying out and becoming brittle. Dry, brittle hair has a tendency to break and fall out very easily.

Incorporating sweet almond oil into your regimen will not only provide your hair with some much-needed nutrition, but it will also ensure that the hair stays strong and grows in faster.

Scalp Massages

Aside from being incredibly relaxing, regular scalp massages (at least 3x a week) can help prevent hair loss as well as encourage healthy hair growth. Massaging the scalp promotes blood flow which provides the scalp with oxygen and other nutrients that are beneficial to maintaining healthy roots. This also encourages a healthy production of sebum-the natural oil produced by the scalp. Although our oil glands shrink gradually as we age, the oil can always be supplemented with other natural oils. Using oils such as castor, lavender, peppermint, or cayenne can heighten the effectiveness of the massage by stimulating the scalp and further increasing the amount of blood flow to the roots of the hair. All the oils mentioned above are excellent for scalp massages.

Caffeine

The biggest benefit caffeine brings to hair is to improve hair growth and structure. Caffeine stimulates and interacts with the hair follicles and even regulates hair growth, so it can promote it and thwart hair loss. You can just keep drinking your morning cup of sunshine to gain that benefit or you can take it a step further (like I do) and enlist in a coffee rinse from time to time to help with hair shedding. I love this easy hair loss remedy!

Here's a breakdown of what you can expect from using it. Caffeine must be applied directly to hair for this benefit (through coffee or tea) which adds shine as well as depth to dark hair. Great for hair butters or conditioners to just add to them to increase hair's natural sheen or shine that many naturals complain their hair is lacking.

Just brew a strong cup of coffee, espresso or black tea (all three are great hair loss remedies) and allow to cool. Pour over your head after you wash and condition. Leave in for 20 minutes and then rinse out. I just pour it over my head after I condition, add my deep conditioner and let the mixture set under my thermal cap for 30 minutes before rinsing out. I LOVE the smell of the coffee mixed with my deep conditioner and feels it gives me and my hair a real pick me up. Check out this coffee oil recipe that is also great for getting that caffeine in for boosting hair growth.

Coffee Oil Hair Growth Recipe

Time to tap into the power of coffee for an excellent hair growth oil recipe. Easy to create and customize, this hair oil can be created using a cold or hot infusion. This oil is great as a pre-poo, scalp massage oil and even a hair serum.

Cold Infusion

What to use:

1 cup pure Olive or Coconut oil

3/4 cup ground coffee

Mason jar

Method:

Combine both ingredients in mason jar. Place the lid on top and shake well. Store for 3 to 4 weeks in a cool dry place shaking it up every single day. Yes, a commitment but worth it! After the end of the 3 to 4 weeks, strain through a cheesecloth or coffee filter and it's ready for use!

<u>Hot Infusion</u>

What to use:

4 tbsp. pure Olive or Coconut oil

8 tbsp. cup ground coffee

Pot or crockpot

Dark glass jar with pump or dropper.

If you want to make a bigger batch, keep the

same formula. Example: 2 cup of ground coffee to 1 cup of oil.

<u>Method:</u>

Combine ground coffee with olive or coconut oil in a pan. Heat over a low heat for at least 30 minutes to a few hours stirring occasionally. If creating a bigger batch, combine ingredients in a small crock pot for a few hours stirring occasionally. Strain the oil using either cheesecloth or a coffee filter.

Cinnamon

As we head over to the sweeter side of combating hair loss, cinnamon or cinnamon powder comes from the bark of tropical, evergreen trees. There are hundreds of types of cinnamon but only four varieties are used for commercial purposes and the main variety is Cassia Cinnamon which is mainly used in the US and Canada. The second most popular variety of cinnamon is is Ceylon Cinnamon which is mostly used in Europe, Mexico and various parts of Asia.

Dermatologist Francesca Fusco, an assistant clinical professor of dermatology at Mount Sinai Hospital in New York, who told Allure Magazine that along with nettle, almond oil, and cayenne, cinnamon is one of the botanicals that's been touted as a follicle stimulator.

Albeit, there are not peer-reviewed research to confirm if there is any truth to these claims she goes on to say, "It would probably help to stimulate blood flow to hair follicles, and that's always a good thing," she says, since "proper circulation is critical to healthy hair growth."

You can also find many woman in the natural hair community who swear by cinnamon as of of their favorite hair loss remedies. While I haven't partaken in any DIY recipes using cinnamon, I agree that any follicle stimulation is a good thing when used properly and in moderation.

Consult a professional

Sometimes we need to bring in the big guns and that means consulting a Dermatologist, MD, Trichologist or professional hairstylist. These professionals can see if your hair loss is attributed to a medical condition, medication or if medicines need to be prescribed to stop the hair loss and to aid in regrowing your hair. Our lifestyle, age, and health can directly affect our hair positively and negatively so consult the professional to ensure you are doing everything possible for healthy scalp and hair.

More Resources

Check out my two hair blogs that have even more information to aid in your hair loss and hair growth problems.

Seriously Natural

Seriously Natural is about Natural hair, beauty and style. From the basics to not so known tidbits; Seriously Natural brings all women the necessities to feel as lovely as they should with proper knowledge, tips and secrets that the experts know! Sharing information on very serious issues surrounding natural hair. I've also sprinkled extras in creativity, news, as well as health issues affecting the Black/African American community.

Natural Hair For Beginners

Natural Hair For Beginners is for women of color who want to go natural but need solid tips to make their journey beautiful and positive. This is where you will get step by step instructions on how to go natural, what you use, when to use it and to ensure you are creating a positive space for your journey.

Thank You!

Thank you for buying the book! I would love for you to leave a review online. Black Women & Hair Loss: How To Stop Losing Our Hair & Gain

Sabrina

Here's a sneak peek of <u>How To Stop Hair Loss in Women</u>, which is now available on Amazon in Kindle and will be in print in April 2018!

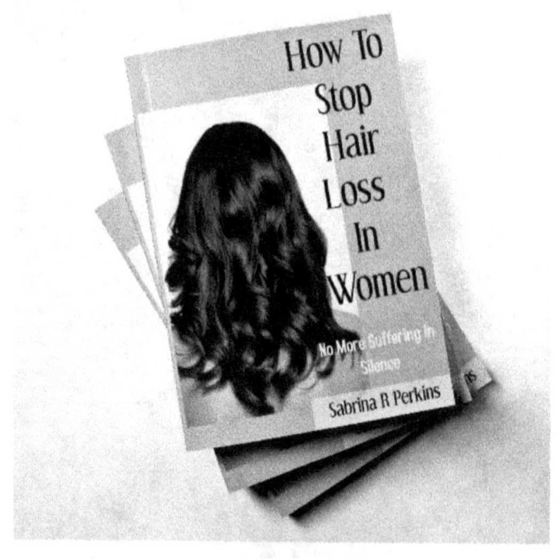

Most women will suffer from some sort of hair loss within her lifetime. From hair thinning to hair fall, women have often thought this was more of a problem for men and does not concern us. Sorry, but many of the very products we've been using over the years have slowly been depleting the hair of its protein and oils that it needs to grow strong and fight off the attack.

Even if the medications you are taking or treatments for certain illnesses are causing the loss of your hair, speaking with a physician is advised because they can offer more natural approaches that have less impact on negatively effecting hair growth.

In 2016, a consumer survey conducted by Keranique® – the Women's Hair Growth Experts™ sheds light on the alarming numbers of American women who have experienced hair loss. According to the survey:

- Nearly 40% of U.S. women 18+ have noticed signs of hair loss or thinning

- Over 50% of US women 58 or older have experienced it

- That number jumps to over 60% for women age 65+

- These signs include: a widening part, hair being thinner than it used to be, significant signs of overall hair loss, and seeing through to the scalp where they couldn't before especially in the temples or at the crown of the head.

What May Be Causing Your Hair Loss

From hair thinning to hair fall, women have often thought this was more of a problem for men and does not concern us. Sorry, but many of the very products we've been using over the years have slowly been depleting the hair of its protein and oils that it needs to grow strong and fight off the attack.

Even if the medications you are taking or treatments for certain illnesses are causing the loss of your hair, speaking with a physician is advised because they can offer more natural approaches that have less impact on hair growth. If you are suffering from above average hair loss and want to take back control of the situation, the following top reasons women suffer from hair loss should help you get a better idea as to what is causing the underlying issue. Check out what are big culprits in women hair loss from the list below.

Anemia

Anemia, simply put is a low iron intake. Not getting enough iron in your diet and couple that with a heavy menstruation flow can cause this problem and this may result in inadequate folic acid.

According to research at WebMD on Anemia, the body begins to produce lower levels of hemoglobin, and that can eventually result in some women suffering from hair loss due to a lack of oxygen to the hair follicles. This makes the hair weaker and easier to break. If the condition persists, hair loss will become more pronounced.

Damaging Hair Practices

For many women, they don't even realize that they are causing their own hair loss as a result of poor hair practices like over processing hair with chemicals from color, hair straightening or perms. Using too much heat, especially without using heat protectants can also weaken the hair and cause breakage or hair loss. Now that weaker and brittle hair is exposed to products with harsh chemicals that further weaker and damage the hair.

Effects of Menopause

One of the things you cannot avoid when it comes to common concern for women and hair loss is how menopause may affect your body. According to Healthline,

> "Research suggests that hair loss during menopause is the result of a hormonal imbalance. Specifically, it's related to a lowered production of estrogen and progesterone. These hormones help hair grow faster and stay on the head for longer periods of time. When the levels of estrogen and progesterone drop, hair grows more slowly and becomes much thinner. A decrease in these hormones also

triggers an increase in the production of androgens, or a group of male hormones. Androgens shrink hair follicles, resulting in hair loss on the head. In some cases, however, these hormones can cause more hair to grow on the face. This is why some menopausal women develop facial "peach fuzz" and small sprouts of hair on the chin."

Powerful Medications

Unfortunately, some of the very medicines we need to stay alive or even just stay healthy can cause subtle to severe hair loss when taking them. Discussing your medications that may cause side effects of hair loss with your doctor is the best way to deal with this issue as there may be alternative meds to try. You are your own advocate so talk to your PCP and see what, if anything, can be done if you sense your hair loss may be due to your meds. Make sure to check out the side effects of your meds as a little research will yield what may be causing this problem.

Extreme Weight Loss

Crash diets, long fasting or just not eating is one of the worst ways to lose weight but they also can cause damage to your body, especially when it comes to your hair. Losing too much weight suddenly may seem attractive but it may be at the expense of your hair. Crash diets deprive the body of those proteins, and that can weaken your strands. When you try to lose too much weight too fast, you are depriving your body of vital nutrients, all of which have a negative impact on hair growth.

The Aging Process

Hair loss can be devastating at any age, but there are ways to prevent it. As we get older, the hair strands weaken causing an increase in breakage and thinning. Usually a result of hormonal changes in the body, the levels of estrogen (which promotes thick hair) we produce begins to decline as we get older. Women also begin to process nutrients less efficiently as we grow older, so diet is crucial to stay healthy and that directly relates to our hair.

www.ingramcontent.com/pod-product-compliance
Lightning Source LLC
Chambersburg PA
CBHW051921250726
48659CB00002B/776